Julius Iseman

CANCER

(Types, Causes and Prevention)

COPYRIGHT STATEMENT

TABLE OF CONTENTS

INTRODUCTION

Cancer, one of the most formidable diseases known to humanity, has captivated the attention of scientists, medical professionals, and individuals worldwide. It is a complex and multifaceted condition characterized by the uncontrolled growth and spread of abnormal cells in the body. This ailment has a profound impact on individuals, families, and societies, making it an ongoing challenge in the field of healthcare.

Cancer can manifest in various forms, affecting different organs and systems within the body. It arises from genetic mutations that alter the normal behavior of cells, leading to their unrestrained division and proliferation. These mutations can be caused by a variety of factors, including environmental influences such as exposure to harmful substances, lifestyle choices like smoking or excessive sun exposure, or even inherent genetic predispositions.

The repercussions of cancer extend beyond the mere presence of abnormal cells. As the disease progresses, it can infiltrate nearby tissues, impair vital organ function, and ultimately spread to distant sites in a process known as metastasis. This invasive nature of cancer poses significant challenges for treatment and management, as it requires comprehensive and personalized approaches to combat the disease effectively.

The impact of cancer reaches far beyond the physical toll it takes on the body. It affects individuals emotionally, mentally, and socially, often causing distress, fear, and uncertainty. Moreover, cancer can strain relationships, disrupt daily routines, and impose financial burdens on those affected. The profound psychological and emotional implications highlight the need for comprehensive support systems and holistic care for cancer patients, as their journey involves not only medical interventions but also psychological and emotional well-being.

Fortunately, immense strides have been made in cancer research over the years. Advances in technology, diagnostics, and treatments have significantly improved outcomes for many patients. New therapies such as targeted therapies, immunotherapies, and precision medicine have revolutionized the field, offering hope for those affected by the disease. Moreover, preventive measures such as early detection screenings and lifestyle modifications have proven effective in reducing the risk of developing certain types of cancer.

CANCER | Julius Iseman

The understanding and management of cancer continue to evolve, with ongoing research striving to unlock its mysteries. Collaboration between scientists, clinicians, and advocacy groups has played a pivotal role in raising awareness, funding research, and improving outcomes. Efforts to enhance public knowledge about prevention, screening, and early detection are essential in reducing the impact of cancer.

Cancer remains a significant global health concern, posing complex challenges for medical professionals, researchers, and society as a whole. It demands continuous progress in diagnosis, treatment, and support systems to alleviate its burden. Although the battle against cancer is far from over, the collective efforts of healthcare professionals, researchers, and individuals affected by this disease provide hope for a future where cancer is better understood, controlled, and ultimately cured.

CHAPTER 1

UNDERSTANDING THE TERM "CANCER"

Cancer is a complex and broad term used to describe a group of diseases characterized by the uncontrolled growth and spread of abnormal cells in the body. It is caused by changes or mutations in the DNA within cells, which disrupt normal cell growth and division processes.

Normally, cells in the body grow, divide, and eventually die in a controlled manner. However, in cancer, these cells undergo genetic changes that allow them to evade the usual checks and balances that regulate cell growth. As a result, they multiply uncontrollably, forming a mass of tissue called a tumor.

Tumors can be either benign or malignant. Benign tumors are non-cancerous and usually do not invade nearby tissues or spread to other parts of the body. On the other hand, malignant tumors are cancerous and have the ability to invade nearby tissues and spread to distant sites through the bloodstream or lymphatic system. This process is known as metastasis.

There are many different types of cancer, each with distinct characteristics, behaviors, and treatment approaches. Some common types include breast cancer, lung cancer, colorectal cancer, prostate cancer, and skin cancer. Each type can have different causes, risk factors, symptoms, and treatment options.

Early detection and treatment are crucial in managing cancer, as it becomes more challenging to treat when it spreads beyond the initial site. Treatment options may include surgery, radiation therapy, chemotherapy, immunotherapy, targeted therapy, hormone therapy, or a combination of these approaches, depending on the type and stage of cancer. Researchers continue to explore new advancements in cancer prevention, diagnosis, and treatment to improve patient outcomes.

TYPES CANCER

There are many different types of cancer, each with its own unique characteristics and affected areas of the body. Here are some common types of cancer:

1. Breast Cancer: This type of cancer usually starts in the breast tissues and can affect both men and women.

2. Lung Cancer: Lung cancer develops in the lungs and is primarily caused by smoking, although it can also occur in non-smokers.

3. Prostate Cancer: Prostate cancer affects the prostate gland in men and is one of the most common types of cancer in males.

4. Colorectal Cancer: This cancer starts in the colon or rectum and usually occurs in older individuals, although it can affect people of all ages.

5. Skin Cancer: There are different types of skin cancer, such as basal cell carcinoma, squamous cell

carcinoma, and melanoma, which are caused by excessive exposure to the sun or UV radiation.

6. Ovarian Cancer: Ovarian cancer affects the ovaries in women and is often difficult to detect in its early stages.

7. Pancreatic Cancer: Pancreatic cancer occurs in the pancreas and is known for its aggressive nature and low survival rates.

8. Leukemia: Leukemia is a cancer of the bone marrow and blood, resulting in the abnormal production of white blood cells.

9. Lymphoma: Lymphoma begins in the lymphatic system, which is responsible for immune function,

and can be classified as Hodgkin's lymphoma or non-Hodgkin's lymphoma.

10. Brain Cancer: Brain tumors can be cancerous or noncancerous and can originate in the brain itself or spread from other parts of the body.

It's important to note that this is not an exhaustive list, as there are many other types of cancer that exist. Awareness, early detection, and regular medical check-ups are crucial in the fight against cancer.

CHAPTER 2

BREAST CANCER

Breast cancer is a type of cancer that develops in the breast cells. It occurs when there is an uncontrolled growth of abnormal cells in the breast tissue. Breast cancer can affect both men and women, although it is predominantly found in women.

There are several risk factors associated with breast cancer, including age, gender, family history, genetic mutations such as BRCA1 and BRCA2, hormonal factors, obesity, alcohol consumption, and exposure to certain chemicals. However, it is important to note that having one or more risk factors does not mean a person will definitely develop breast cancer, as many individuals with no known risk factors still develop the disease.

Early detection plays a crucial role in improving breast cancer outcomes. Regular breast self-examinations, clinical breast examinations by a healthcare provider, and mammograms are important screening methods that can help detect breast cancer at an early stage.

Symptoms of breast cancer may include a lump or thickening in the breast or underarm area, changes in breast size or shape, skin dimpling or puckering, nipple abnormalities such as inversion or discharge, and redness or scaling of the breast skin. It's important to note that these symptoms can also be caused by conditions other than breast cancer, so it's best to consult a healthcare professional for proper evaluation if any concerns arise.

If breast cancer is suspected, various diagnostic tests may be performed, such as mammograms, ultrasounds, MRI scans, and biopsies. Treatment options for breast cancer typically involve a combination of surgery, radiation therapy, chemotherapy, targeted therapy, and hormone therapy. The specific treatment plan depends on factors such as the stage of cancer, the type of breast cancer, and individual patient factors.

Support and care for individuals with breast cancer extend beyond medical treatment. Emotional support, counseling, support groups, and access to resources can greatly assist patients and their families throughout the treatment and recovery process.

While breast cancer remains a significant health challenge, advances in research, early detection, and treatment have improved survival rates over the years. It's essential to stay informed about breast health and to

CANCER | Julius Iseman

consult healthcare professionals for routine screenings and any concerns regarding breast health.

CAUSES OF BREAST CANCER

Breast cancer is a complex disease, and the exact causes are not fully understood. However, there are several known factors that can increase the risk of developing breast cancer. Here are some possible causes:

1. Age: The risk of breast cancer increases as a person gets older. Most cases of breast cancer occur in women over the age of 50.

2. Gender: Breast cancer is much more common in women than men. Although men can also develop breast cancer, it is rare.

3. Family history and genetics: Certain gene mutations, such as BRCA1 and BRCA2, can be inherited and significantly increase the risk of breast cancer. Having a close family member, like a mother or sister, with breast cancer may also increase the risk.

4. Hormonal factors: Estrogen and progesterone, hormones that regulate the menstrual cycle, may play a role in the development of breast cancer. Factors such as early onset of menstruation (before age 12) or late menopause (after age 55) can increase the risk. Also, having the first child after the age of 35 or never having children may be associated with a higher risk.

5. Previous history of breast cancer or certain benign breast conditions: Women who have had breast cancer before are at a higher risk of developing it again. Additionally, certain types of benign breast conditions, such as atypical hyperplasia, may increase the risk.

6. Lifestyle factors: Certain lifestyle choices may increase the risk of breast cancer, such as excessive alcohol consumption, smoking, obesity, and a sedentary lifestyle. A high-fat diet may also contribute to the risk.

7. Radiation exposure: Previous exposure to radiation, especially at a young age, may increase the risk of developing breast cancer later in life.

It's important to note that having one or more of these risk factors doesn't necessarily mean a person will develop breast cancer, while the absence of risk factors does not guarantee safety. Regular screenings and early detection are crucial in identifying breast cancer at its early stages when treatment is often more effective. If you have concerns about breast cancer, it's best to consult with a healthcare professional.

PREVENTION OF BREAST CANCER

Prevention of breast cancer involves several strategies that can help reduce the risk of developing the disease. Here are some key measures:

1. Regular Breast Self-Exams: Perform monthly breast self-exams to become familiar with your breasts' normal look and feel. Any changes, such as new lumps or abnormalities, should be reported to your healthcare provider promptly.

2. Clinical Breast Exams: Have regular clinical breast exams conducted by a healthcare professional. They can help detect any potential signs or symptoms of breast cancer.

3. Mammograms: Schedule regular mammograms as recommended by your healthcare provider. Mammography is an effective screening tool for detecting breast cancer early, especially in women

over the age of 40 or those at higher risk.

4. Lifestyle Choices: Adopting a healthy lifestyle can significantly reduce the risk of breast cancer. This includes maintaining a balanced diet rich in fruits, vegetables, whole grains, and lean proteins. Avoid excessive alcohol consumption, limit processed and red meat intake, and avoid or quit smoking.

5. Physical Activity: Engage in regular physical activity and aim for a minimum of 150 minutes of moderate aerobic activity or 75 minutes of vigorous aerobic activity each week. Physical exercise can help reduce the risk of breast cancer.

6. Maintain a Healthy Weight: Strive for a healthy weight by maintaining a balanced diet and participating in regular physical activity. Obesity and excess body fat have been linked to an increased risk of breast cancer, especially after menopause.

7. Breastfeeding: For mothers who can and choose to breastfeed, there is evidence suggesting it may have a protective effect against breast cancer. Breastfeeding for at least several months can provide benefits for both the mother and child.

8. Hormone Therapy: If you're considering hormonal therapy for menopause symptoms, discuss the potential risks and benefits with your healthcare provider. Prolonged use

of combined hormone replacement therapy (estrogen and progestin) may increase the risk of breast cancer in some women.

9. Genetic Testing and Counseling: If you have a family history of breast cancer or other risk factors, consider genetic testing to determine if you carry any known gene mutations associated with the disease. Genetic counseling can help assess your risk and guide appropriate preventive measures.

10. Stay Informed: Stay up to date with the latest research and recommendations by consulting your healthcare provider or reputable organizations like the American

Cancer Society or the National Breast Cancer Foundation.

Remember, while these measures can help reduce the risk of breast cancer, they do not guarantee prevention. Regular screenings and early detection remain critical for effective management and treatment of breast cancer.

CHAPTER 3

LUNG CANCER

Lung cancer is a type of cancer that starts in the cells of the lungs. It is one of the most common forms of cancer and a leading cause of cancer-related deaths worldwide. Lung cancer can be broadly categorized into two main types: non-small cell lung cancer (NSCLC) and small cell lung cancer (SCLC).

NSCLC is the most common type, accounting for about 85% of all lung cancer cases. It includes subtypes such as adenocarcinoma, squamous cell carcinoma, and large cell carcinoma. SCLC, on the other hand, is a more aggressive and rapidly growing form of lung cancer, typically associated with smoking.

The primary cause of lung cancer is cigarette smoking, with around 85% of cases attributed to smoking. However, non-smokers can also develop lung cancer, usually due to exposure to secondhand smoke, environmental pollution, radon gas, certain industrial chemicals, or a family history of the disease.

Symptoms of lung cancer can vary but may include a persistent cough, chest pain, coughing up blood, wheezing, shortness of breath, fatigue, unexplained weight loss, and recurrent respiratory infections. However, it's important to note that not everyone with lung cancer experiences noticeable symptoms in the early stages.

Early detection is crucial for improving the prognosis of lung cancer. Diagnostic tests for lung cancer may include imaging scans like chest X-rays, CT scans, or MRI scans, as well as sputum cytology, biopsy, or bronchoscopy.

Treatment options for lung cancer depend on several factors, including the type and stage of the cancer and the patient's overall health. Common treatments may involve surgery to remove the tumor, chemotherapy, radiation therapy, targeted therapy, immunotherapy, or a combination of these approaches.

Prevention plays a vital role in reducing the risk of developing lung cancer. The most effective way to prevent lung cancer is to avoid smoking or to quit smoking if you are already a smoker. Additionally, minimizing exposure to secondhand smoke, industrial pollutants, or other harmful airborne substances is important.

If you suspect any symptoms or have concerns about lung cancer, it is advisable to consult a healthcare professional for a proper diagnosis and appropriate treatment options.

CAUSES OF LUNG CANCER

There are several possible causes of lung cancer, including:

1. Tobacco smoke: Smoking cigarettes, cigars, or pipes is the leading cause of lung cancer. The harmful chemicals found in tobacco smoke can damage the cells lining the lungs and lead to the development of cancer.

2. Secondhand smoke: Exposure to secondhand smoke, which is the

smoke emitted by a smoker and inhaled by others, can also increase the risk of developing lung cancer.

3. Radon gas: Radon is a naturally occurring radioactive gas that can be found in homes and buildings. Prolonged exposure to high levels of radon gas can increase the risk of lung cancer, especially in those who smoke.

4. Occupational exposure: Certain occupations, such as construction, mining, manufacturing, and transportation, involve exposure to carcinogens like asbestos, diesel exhaust, arsenic, and certain chemicals. Prolonged exposure to these substances over time can

increase the risk of developing lung cancer.

5. Air pollution: Long-term exposure to air pollution, particularly in highly polluted areas, can contribute to the development of lung cancer. Fine particles and toxic substances present in the air can be inhaled into the lungs and cause damage over time.

6. Genetic factors: Some people may have an inherited predisposition to developing lung cancer. Certain genetic mutations and family history of lung cancer can increase the risk.

7. Previous history of lung diseases: Individuals with a history of lung diseases, such as chronic obstructive pulmonary disease (COPD) or

tuberculosis, may have an increased risk of developing lung cancer.

It's important to note that while these factors can increase the risk of developing lung cancer, not everyone exposed to them will develop the disease. Quitting smoking, reducing exposure to environmental pollutants, and adopting a healthy lifestyle can help reduce the risk of lung cancer. Regular check-ups and screenings may also help with early detection and treatment.

PREVENTION OF LUNG CANCER

Prevention of lung cancer involves adopting certain lifestyle choices and avoiding exposure to risk factors that are known to increase the likelihood of developing the disease. Here are some key prevention strategies:

1. Quit Smoking: Smoking is the leading cause of lung cancer, accounting for about 85% of cases. If you're a smoker, quitting is the most effective way to prevent lung cancer. Seek support from healthcare professionals, use medications, join support groups, or try nicotine replacement therapy to help you quit.

2. Avoid Secondhand Smoke: Secondhand smoke is a significant risk factor for lung cancer. Avoid environments where people smoke, and encourage family members, friends, and co-workers to not smoke around you or in your living space.

3. Radon Gas: Radon is a naturally occurring radioactive gas that can seep into homes and buildings through cracks in the foundation. It is the second leading cause of lung cancer and is responsible for about 10% of cases. Test your home for radon and take appropriate measures to reduce its levels if necessary.

4. Occupational Hazards: Exposure to certain workplace substances like asbestos, arsenic, diesel exhaust, uranium, and some chemicals can increase the risk of lung cancer. Follow safety protocols, use protective equipment, and minimize exposure to such substances if you work in a high-risk industry.

5. Environmental Pollution: Limit exposure to outdoor air pollution and indoor pollutants like cooking fumes, mold, and volatile organic compounds (VOCs) from household products. Ensure proper ventilation in your home and workspaces and use air purifiers if necessary.

6. Healthy Diet: Eat a balanced diet rich in vegetables, fruits, whole grains, and lean proteins. Antioxidant-rich foods may help reduce the risk of cancer. Avoid excessive consumption of processed meats, which have been linked to an increased risk of lung cancer.

7. Physical Activity: Engage in regular physical activity to improve overall health. Exercise has been shown to

lower the risk of cancer, including lung cancer. Aim for at least 150 minutes of moderate-intensity aerobic activity or 75 minutes of vigorous-intensity activity per week.

8. Genetic Counseling: If there is a family history of lung cancer or other genetic factors that increase your risk, consider genetic counseling to understand your individual risk profile and appropriate preventive measures.

Remember, while these prevention strategies can reduce the risk of lung cancer, they do not guarantee complete protection. Regular screenings and early detection are crucial for individuals at higher risk or with a history of exposure to carcinogens. Consult with a healthcare professional for personalized advice based on your specific risk factors.

CHAPTER 4

PROSTATE CANCER

Prostate cancer is a type of cancer that occurs in the prostate gland, a small walnut-shaped gland in men that produces seminal fluid. It is one of the most common types of cancer among men, particularly those who are older.

The exact cause of prostate cancer is unknown, but various risk factors have been identified. Age is the primary risk factor, with the likelihood of developing prostate cancer increasing significantly after the age of 50. Other risk factors include a family history of the disease, certain genetic mutations, and race (prostate cancer is more common in African American men).

In the early stages, prostate cancer may not cause noticeable symptoms. However, as the disease progresses, symptoms may include difficulty urinating, weak urine flow, frequent urination (especially at night), blood in the urine or semen, erectile dysfunction, pain or discomfort in the pelvic area, and bone pain.

If prostate cancer is suspected, a physician may perform various diagnostic tests, including a digital rectal exam (DRE), prostate-specific antigen (PSA) blood test, and possibly a biopsy. These tests help determine the presence, stage, and aggressiveness of the cancer.

Treatment options for prostate cancer depend on various factors such as the stage of the cancer, the age and overall health of the patient, and individual preferences.

Treatment options may include active surveillance (regular monitoring without immediate treatment), surgery, radiation therapy, hormone therapy, chemotherapy, or immunotherapy. The choice of treatment is typically made in consultation with a healthcare team and may involve a multidisciplinary approach.

Regular prostate cancer screening is often recommended for men at higher risk, enabling early detection and improving the chances of successful treatment. However, the decision to undergo screening should be based on individual risk factors and should be discussed with a healthcare provider.

It's important to note that while prostate cancer can be serious, many cases are slow-growing and may not require immediate treatment. Each case is unique, and a thorough evaluation by medical professionals is crucial in determining the appropriate course of action.

CAUSES OF PROSTATE CANCER

Prostate cancer is a complex disease with multiple contributing factors. While the exact cause of prostate cancer is still unknown, several factors have been identified that increase the risk of developing the disease. Here are some possible causes and risk factors associated with prostate cancer:

1. Age: Prostate cancer is more common in older men. The risk of developing prostate cancer increases significantly after the age of 50.

2. Family history: Having a family history of prostate cancer, particularly in first-degree relatives (such as a father or brother), increases the risk. Genetic factors may contribute to the development of prostate cancer.

3. Genetics: Certain inherited gene mutations, such as mutations in the BRCA1 and BRCA2 genes, have been linked to an increased risk of developing prostate cancer.

4. Race and ethnicity: Prostate cancer is more prevalent in certain ethnic groups, particularly among African American men. They have a higher risk of developing prostate cancer and are more likely to be diagnosed at an advanced stage.

CANCER | Julius Iseman

5. Hormonal factors: Testosterone, the male sex hormone, plays a role in the growth and function of the prostate gland. Higher levels of testosterone or other hormonal imbalances may be associated with an increased risk of prostate cancer.

6. Diet and lifestyle: A diet high in red meat and high-fat dairy products, as well as a sedentary lifestyle, may contribute to the development of prostate cancer. Consuming a diet rich in fruits and vegetables, maintaining a healthy weight, and engaging in regular physical activity may help reduce the risk.

7. Smoking: Although the direct link is not fully understood, smoking has been associated with an increased

CANCER | Julius Iseman

risk of aggressive forms of prostate cancer and worse treatment outcomes.

8. Exposure to certain chemicals: Occupational exposure to certain chemicals, such as cadmium or Agent Orange, may increase the risk of developing prostate cancer. However, the evidence for these associations is limited.

It's important to note that having one or more of these risk factors does not necessarily mean an individual will develop prostate cancer. Conversely, some individuals may develop prostate cancer without exhibiting any of these risk factors. Regular prostate cancer screening and discussions with healthcare professionals can help individuals understand their specific risk and take appropriate steps for prevention or early detection.

PREVENTION OF PROSTATE CANCER

Prevention of prostate cancer involves adopting a proactive approach aimed at reducing the risk factors associated with the development of the disease. While there is no guaranteed way to prevent prostate cancer, certain lifestyle modifications and risk reduction strategies can help lower the chances of developing the condition. Here are some recommendations for the prevention of prostate cancer:

1. Eat a healthy diet: Consuming a diet rich in fruits, vegetables, whole grains, and lean proteins is beneficial

for overall health, including prostate health. Include foods such as tomatoes, cruciferous vegetables (broccoli, cauliflower, cabbage), berries, nuts, and fish like salmon that are high in omega-3 fatty acids.

2. Limit red meat and processed foods: A high intake of red and processed meats has been associated with an increased risk of prostate cancer. Limit your consumption of these foods and opt for healthier protein sources like poultry, fish, beans, and lentils.

3. Maintain a healthy weight: Obesity or being overweight has been linked to an increased risk of developing prostate cancer. Engage in regular

physical activity and maintain a healthy weight to reduce your risk.

4. Engage in regular exercise: Regular exercise, such as brisk walking, jogging, swimming, or cycling, has been shown to have a protective effect against prostate cancer. Aim for at least 150 minutes of moderate-intensity exercise or 75 minutes of vigorous-intensity exercise each week.

5. Get screened: Although routine prostate cancer screening is not universally recommended, it is important to discuss with your doctor when and how often you should be screened based on your age, risk factors, and family history.

6. Limit alcohol consumption: Heavy alcohol consumption has been associated with an increased risk of prostate cancer. If you choose to drink alcohol, do so in moderation - up to one drink per day for men.

7. Quit smoking: Smoking has been linked to several types of cancer, including prostate cancer. Quitting smoking is not only beneficial for prostate health but overall well-being.

8. Maintain a healthy lifestyle: Adopting a healthy lifestyle overall, including getting enough sleep, managing stress levels, and avoiding environmental toxins, can contribute to reducing the risk of prostate cancer.

CANCER | Julius Iseman

It's important to note that while these strategies can help reduce the risk of prostate cancer, they may not guarantee complete prevention. Regular check-ups, awareness of any symptoms, and discussing concerns with a healthcare professional are crucial for early detection and appropriate management of prostate cancer.

CHAPTER 5

COLORECTAL CANCER

Colorectal cancer, also known as bowel cancer or colon cancer, is a type of cancer that affects the colon or rectum. It is one of the most common types of cancer worldwide. Colorectal cancer typically begins as a small polyp, which is a noncancerous growth, on the inner lining of the colon or rectum. Over time, some polyps can develop into cancer.

CAUSES OF COLORECTAL CANCER

The exact cause of colorectal cancer is unknown, but several risk factors have been identified. These include:

1. Age: The risk of developing colorectal cancer increases as you get older, with most cases occurring in individuals over 50.

2. Family history: Having a close relative, such as a parent or sibling, with colorectal cancer increases your risk.

3. Personal history of polyps or inflammatory bowel disease: If you have previously had colorectal polyps or inflammatory bowel disease, you are at a higher risk.

4. Lifestyle factors: A diet high in red and processed meats, low in fiber, lack of physical activity, smoking, and excessive alcohol consumption can increase the risk.

Symptoms:

Colorectal cancer often does not cause symptoms in its early stages, which is why routine screening is essential. However, as the disease progresses, the following symptoms may occur:

1) Change in bowel habits, such as persistent diarrhea or constipation.

2) Blood in the stool or rectal bleeding.

3) Abdominal pain or discomfort.

4) Unexplained weight loss.

5) Fatigue and weakness.

6) Nausea or vomiting.

PREVENTION OF COLORECTAL CANCER

Early detection through screening is crucial in preventing colorectal cancer or catching it at an early stage when it is more treatable. Common screening methods include:

1. Colonoscopy: A procedure where a flexible tube with a camera is inserted into the rectum and colon to examine the entire colon and remove any polyps.

2. Fecal occult blood test (FOBT): A test that checks for hidden blood in the stool, which can indicate the presence of polyps or cancer.

3. Flexible sigmoidoscopy: Similar to a colonoscopy, but it only examines the lower part of the colon.

Treatment:

Treatment for colorectal cancer depends on several factors, including the stage of the cancer, location, and overall health of the individual. Treatment options may include:

1. Surgery: The most common approach is surgical removal of the tumor and nearby lymph nodes.

2. Chemotherapy: Medications can be used to kill cancer cells or stop their growth.

3. Radiation therapy: High-energy rays are directed at the cancer cells to destroy them or prevent their growth.

4. Targeted therapy: Drugs are designed to target specific abnormalities in cancer cells to inhibit their growth.

It is important to consult with healthcare professionals for personalized advice, treatment options, and regular screening recommendations based on your individual circumstances and risk factors.

CHAPTER 6

SKIN CANCER

Skin cancer is a type of cancer that begins in the skin cells. It occurs when there is an abnormal growth of skin cells, usually due to damage or mutation in their DNA. The most common cause of skin cancer is excessive exposure to ultraviolet (UV) radiation from the sun or tanning beds.

There are several types of skin cancer, with the most common ones being basal cell carcinoma (BCC), squamous cell carcinoma (SCC), and melanoma. BCC and SCC are more common but are generally less aggressive, while melanoma is less common but more dangerous.

Early detection and treatment of skin cancer are crucial for better outcomes.

Dermatologists are trained to diagnose and treat skin cancer by conducting a thorough examination and may perform a biopsy if necessary. Regular self-examination of the skin can also help detect any changes or abnormalities that may indicate skin cancer.

Prevention of skin cancer involves taking steps to protect the skin from harmful UV radiation. These measures include wearing protective clothing, using a broad-spectrum sunscreen with a high SPF, seeking shade during peak sunlight hours, and avoiding tanning beds.

It's important to stay informed about the risk factors, symptoms, and preventive measures related to skin cancer. If you notice any unusual changes in your skin, such as the appearance of new moles, changes in existing moles, or growths that don't heal, it's important to consult a healthcare professional for further evaluation.

CAUSES OF SKIN CANCER

Skin cancer is primarily caused by exposure to ultraviolet (UV) radiation from the sun or artificial sources such as tanning beds. The following are some key factors and causes that contribute to the development of skin cancer:

1. Sun exposure: Excessive and unprotected exposure to the sun's UV rays is the leading cause of skin cancer. Prolonged exposure over time damages the DNA within the skin cells, leading to abnormal growth and the formation of cancerous cells.

2. Tanning beds: Artificial sources of UV radiation, such as tanning beds and sunlamps, also increase the risk of skin cancer. The concentrated UV exposure from these devices can be particularly harmful, especially when used in excess or from a young age.

3. Fair skin tone: People with fair skin, light hair color, and light eye color are more susceptible to skin damage from UV radiation. The lower level of melanin (the pigment responsible for skin color) in fair skin offers less protection against the sun's harmful rays.

4. Family history: Having a family history of skin cancer increases the risk. Certain inherited gene mutations, such as those found in

familial melanoma, can enhance a person's susceptibility to developing skin cancer.

5. Age: The risk of skin cancer increases with age. The cumulative exposure to UV radiation throughout life can have a greater impact on older individuals.

6. Previous skin cancer: If you have had skin cancer before, you have a higher chance of developing it again in the future. Regular skin check-ups and monitoring are essential for early detection and treatment.

7. Weakened immune system: A weak immune system can make it more difficult for the body to fight off cancerous cells. Conditions such as HIV/AIDS, organ transplant

recipients taking immunosuppressant medications, or those with certain autoimmune diseases are at a higher risk.

8. Certain moles or skin conditions: People with many moles (especially atypical mole syndrome) or certain pre-existing skin conditions may have an increased risk of developing skin cancer.

9. Occupational exposure: Some occupations involve prolonged outdoor work and increased sun exposure. Farmers, construction workers, lifeguards, and outdoor recreational workers are examples of professions that may face an elevated risk.

It's important to note that while these factors increase the risk of developing skin cancer, they do not guarantee its occurrence. Taking preventative measures and protecting your skin from UV rays through practices like wearing sunscreen, protective clothing, and seeking shade can help lower the risk. Regular skin examinations and early detection are crucial for successful treatment outcomes.

PREVENTION OF SKIN CANCER

Prevention of skin cancer involves adopting various strategies to minimize the risk of developing the disease. Here are some key steps you can take to protect your skin:

1. Limit exposure to ultraviolet (UV) radiation: UV radiation from the sun

is the primary risk factor for skin cancer. Take the following precautions to reduce exposure:

a. Seek shade: Avoid spending long periods in direct sunlight, especially during peak hours between 10 a.m. and 4 p.m.

b. Wear protective clothing: Cover your skin as much as possible with lightweight, loose-fitting, long-sleeved shirts, pants, wide-brimmed hats, and sunglasses that block both UVA and UVB rays.

c. Apply sunscreen: Use broad-spectrum sunscreen with a sun protection factor (SPF) of 30 or higher on all exposed skin, even on cloudy days. Reapply every two hours or after swimming or sweating.

2. Avoid indoor tanning: Tanning beds and sunlamps emit UV radiation, which significantly increases the risk of skin cancer. It is best to avoid these artificial sources of UV exposure.

3. Perform regular self-exams: Conduct monthly self-examinations of your skin to monitor any changes in moles, birthmarks, or other spots. Look for any new growths, changes in color, size, shape, or texture, as well as any spot that itches, bleeds, or is not healing. If you notice any concerning developments, consult a dermatologist.

4. Get professional skin examinations: Regular full-body skin examinations by a dermatologist can help identify any early signs of skin cancer. Discuss with your doctor about the recommended frequency of appointments based on your risk factors.

5. Be aware of your personal risk factors: Some people are at higher risk for developing skin cancer, including those with fair skin, a history of sunburns, a family history of skin cancer, a weakened immune system, or a large number of moles. If you have any personal risk factors, take extra precautions and consider discussing them with a healthcare professional.

Remember, prevention is vital but early detection is equally important. If you notice any suspicious changes on your skin, it's crucial to seek medical evaluation promptly.

CHAPTER 7

OVARIAN CANCER

Ovarian cancer is a type of cancer that begins in the ovaries, the reproductive organs responsible for producing eggs and hormones. It is the fifth most common cancer among women worldwide and often goes undetected until it has progressed to an advanced stage.

Risk factors for ovarian cancer include age (it is more common in older women), family history of ovarian or breast cancer, certain genetic mutations (such as BRCA1 and BRCA2), hormone replacement therapy, obesity, and a personal history of breast, colorectal, or endometrial cancer.

Symptoms of ovarian cancer can be vague and may overlap with other conditions, making early diagnosis challenge. Some common signs include abdominal bloating or swelling, pelvic pain, feeling full quickly while eating, persistent indigestion, changes in bowel or bladder habits, unexplained weight loss or gain, fatigue, and changes in menstrual patterns.

If you experience persistent or unusual symptoms, it is important to consult a healthcare professional. They may perform a physical examination, order blood tests (such as CA-125), and recommend imaging tests like ultrasound, CT scan, or MRI to evaluate the ovaries.

Treatment options for ovarian cancer depend on the stage and spread of the disease. Surgery is typically the first step and involves removing the ovaries, fallopian tubes, and the uterus in some cases.

Chemotherapy may also be recommended to destroy remaining cancer cells and prevent their recurrence. In advanced cases, targeted therapy or radiation therapy might be used.

Supportive care is an essential part of ovarian cancer treatment, focusing on managing side effects, providing emotional support, and improving quality of life. It is important for patients to have a multidisciplinary healthcare team that includes oncologists, surgeons, nurses, and other specialists working together to develop an appropriate treatment plan.

Research and awareness efforts continue to improve early detection and treatment options for ovarian cancer. It is crucial for women to be proactive about their health, attend regular check-ups, be familiar with their bodies, and seek medical attention if they experience any persistent or concerning symptoms.

CAUSES OF OVARIAN CANCER

Ovarian cancer is a complex disease, and the exact causes are not fully understood. However, several factors have been identified as potential contributors to the development of ovarian cancer. Here are some of the known causes and risk factors:

1. Age: The risk of developing ovarian cancer increases with age, particularly after menopause. Most cases are diagnosed in women over the age of 50.

2. Family history: If you have a close relative (such as a mother, sister, or daughter) who has had ovarian cancer, your risk of developing the

disease is higher. Certain inherited gene mutations, such as BRCA1 and BRCA2, significantly increase the risk of ovarian cancer.

3. Personal history of cancer: Women who have had breast, colorectal, or uterine cancer are at a higher risk of developing ovarian cancer.

4. Hormonal factors: Factors that affect the number of times a woman ovulates, such as early onset of menstruation, late menopause, and infertility, can increase the risk of ovarian cancer. Having children at a later age or never having children also plays a role.

5. Endometriosis: Women who have been diagnosed with endometriosis, a condition where the tissue lining

the uterus grows outside of it, may have an increased risk of ovarian cancer.

6. Obesity: Being overweight or obese is associated with a higher risk of developing ovarian cancer.

7. Hormone replacement therapy (HRT): Long-term use of estrogen-alone hormone replacement therapy (HRT) after menopause may increase the risk of ovarian cancer.

8. Smoking: Smoking has been linked to a small increased risk of developing certain types of ovarian cancer.

It's important to note that having one or more of these risk factors does not mean a person will develop ovarian cancer. Many women without any known risk factors can still develop the disease, while some with several risk factors may never develop it. Proper screening, early detection, and regular conversations with healthcare professionals are vital for proper prevention and management of ovarian cancer.

PREVENTION OF OVARIAN CANCER

Prevention of ovarian cancer involves several strategies that can help reduce the risk of developing the disease. Although it's not possible to completely eliminate the risk of ovarian cancer, taking proactive steps can make a difference. Here are some recommendations for ovarian cancer prevention:

CANCER | Julius Iseman

1. Birth Control Pills: Taking oral contraceptives (birth control pills) can reduce the risk of ovarian cancer. Women who use birth control pills for five or more years have a lower chance of developing this type of cancer.

2. Pregnancy and Breastfeeding: Being pregnant and breastfeeding can lower the risk of ovarian cancer. The more pregnancies and lactation periods a woman has, the lower her risk may be.

3. Tubal Ligation or Hysterectomy: Surgical procedures like tubal ligation, which involves blocking or sealing the fallopian tubes, or hysterectomy, which involves removing the uterus, can

significantly reduce the risk of ovarian cancer.

4. Genetic Testing and Counseling: If there is a strong family history of ovarian or breast cancer, it is important to consider genetic testing for gene mutations, such as BRCA1 and BRCA2. Genetic counseling can help individuals understand their risk and make informed decisions regarding preventive measures.

5. Lifestyle Factors: Adopting a healthy lifestyle can indirectly reduce the risk of ovarian cancer. This includes regular exercise, maintaining a healthy weight, eating a balanced diet rich in fruits and vegetables, and avoiding tobacco and excessive alcohol consumption.

6. Awareness and Regular Health Check-ups: Staying informed about the signs and symptoms of ovarian cancer is crucial. Pay attention to any changes in your menstrual cycle, abdominal or pelvic pain, bloating, and frequent urination. Regular check-ups and screenings can help with early detection and treatment.

It is important to note that these prevention strategies may not be feasible or appropriate for everyone. Consult with your healthcare provider to assess your individual risk factors and determine the best prevention plan for you.

CHAPTER 8

PANCREATIC CANCER

Pancreatic cancer is a type of cancer that affects the pancreas, a gland located deep within the abdomen. The pancreas plays a crucial role in digestion and regulating blood sugar levels by producing digestive enzymes and hormones such as insulin.

Pancreatic cancer occurs when abnormal cells in the pancreas begin to divide and grow uncontrollably, forming a tumor. It is a relatively rare form of cancer but is known for its aggressive nature and tendency to spread rapidly to other parts of the body.

The exact cause of pancreatic cancer is not fully understood, but certain risk factors have been identified. These include age (most cases occur in people over 65), smoking, obesity, a family history of pancreatic cancer or certain genetic syndromes, chronic pancreatitis (inflammation of the pancreas), and diabetes.

Unfortunately, pancreatic cancer is often difficult to detect in its early stages. Symptoms typically do not appear until the disease has advanced, and they can vary depending on the location and size of the tumor. Common signs and symptoms include abdominal or back pain, unintentional weight loss, jaundice (yellowing of the skin and eyes), loss of appetite, fatigue, and digestive issues.

If pancreatic cancer is suspected, various diagnostic tests may be performed, such as imaging tests (CT scan, MRI, ultrasound), blood tests to measure certain biomarkers, and sometimes a biopsy to examine a small sample of the tumor tissue for further analysis.

The treatment for pancreatic cancer depends on several factors, including the stage of the cancer, the location and size of the tumor, as well as the patient's overall health. Treatment options may include surgery to remove the tumor, chemotherapy, radiation therapy, targeted therapy, immunotherapy, or a combination of these approaches.

Unfortunately, pancreatic cancer has a generally poor prognosis. This is due to factors such as late detection, aggressive nature, and a lack of effective treatment options for advanced stages. The high mortality rate associated with pancreatic cancer highlights the importance of early detection and ongoing research efforts to improve diagnosis, treatment, and patient outcomes.

If you or someone you know has concerns about pancreatic cancer or any health-related issue, it is important to consult with a qualified healthcare professional who can provide appropriate guidance and support.

CAUSES OF PANCREATIC CANCER

Pancreatic cancer occurs when abnormal cells in the pancreas start to multiply and form a tumor. While the exact cause of pancreatic cancer is unknown, there are certain risk factors that can increase the likelihood of developing this disease. Here are some of the factors that are associated with pancreatic cancer:

1. Age: Pancreatic cancer is more common in older adults, with the majority of cases occurring in people over the age of 65.

2. Smoking: Cigarette smoking is one of the most significant risk factors for pancreatic cancer. Smokers are two times more likely to develop the disease than non-smokers.

3. Family history: Having a close relative, such as a parent, sibling, or child, diagnosed with pancreatic cancer increases the risk. Certain genetic syndromes, such as hereditary pancreatitis, may also contribute to the development of this cancer.

4. Obesity: Being overweight or obese is linked to an increased risk of

pancreatic cancer. It is believed to be due to higher levels of insulin, a hormone that may promote the growth of cancer cells.

5. Diabetes: People with long-standing diabetes have a higher risk of developing pancreatic cancer. However, the relationship between the two is complex and not entirely understood.

6. Chronic pancreatitis: Inflammation of the pancreas over a long period of time (chronic pancreatitis) can increase the risk of developing pancreatic cancer. Chronic pancreatitis may be caused by heavy alcohol use, certain inherited conditions, or due to other factors.

7. Diet: Some studies suggest that a diet high in red and processed meats, as well as low in fruits and vegetables, may contribute to the development of pancreatic cancer. However, more research is needed to confirm this relationship.

It's important to note that having one or more risk factors does not mean that a person will definitely develop pancreatic cancer, as many people with the disease have no identifiable risk factors. Additionally, there may be individuals who develop pancreatic cancer without any known risk factors. If you have concerns about your risk or symptoms related to pancreatic cancer, it is advisable to consult with a healthcare professional.

PREVENTION OF PANCREATIC CANCER

Pancreatic cancer is a serious condition that requires attention to preventive measures. While it's not always possible to prevent pancreatic cancer from developing, there are certain lifestyle choices that can reduce your risk. Here are some strategies you can follow:

1. Don't smoke: Smoking is one of the leading causes of pancreatic cancer. If you smoke, consider quitting as soon as possible. If you're a non-smoker, be sure to avoid secondhand smoke exposure.

2. Eat a healthy diet: Focus on consuming a diet rich in fruits, vegetables, whole grains, and lean proteins. Limit your intake of red

and processed meats, as these have been associated with a higher risk of pancreatic cancer.

3. Maintain a healthy weight: Obesity and being overweight are risk factors for many types of cancer, including pancreatic cancer. Engage in regular physical activity and try to maintain a healthy body weight.

4. Limit alcohol consumption: Excessive alcohol consumption is a risk factor for pancreatic cancer. It is advised to limit alcohol intake to moderate levels — up to one drink per day for women and up to two drinks per day for men.

5. Stay hydrated: Drinking an adequate amount of water and staying

hydrated is vital for overall health, including the health of your pancreas.

6. Regular exercise: Engaging in regular physical activity can contribute to maintaining a healthy weight, reducing inflammation, and improving overall well-being. Aim for at least 150 minutes of moderate-intensity exercise per week.

7. Be vigilant with your health: Attend regular check-ups and screenings as recommended by your healthcare provider. If you have a family history of pancreatic cancer or any other risk factors, discuss it with your doctor, who may suggest additional screenings or surveillance.

It's worth noting that while these preventative strategies can reduce your risk of pancreatic cancer, they do not guarantee complete prevention. It's essential to be aware of the early signs and symptoms of pancreatic cancer and seek medical attention promptly if you notice any concerns.

CHAPTER 9

LEUKEMIA

Leukemia is a type of cancer that affects the body's blood-forming tissues, including the bone marrow and the lymphatic system. It involves the uncontrolled production of abnormal white blood cells, which crowd out healthy blood cells and impair the body's ability to fight infections.

There are several types of leukemia, classified based on the specific type of white blood cells affected and the rate of disease progression. The main types include acute lymphoblastic leukemia (ALL), acute myeloid leukemia (AML), chronic lymphocytic leukemia (CLL), and chronic myeloid leukemia (CML).

The exact cause of leukemia is not known in most cases, but certain risk factors can increase the likelihood of developing the disease. These include radiation exposure, certain genetic conditions, hereditary factors, exposure to certain chemicals and toxins, and previous chemotherapy or radiation treatment for other cancers.

The symptoms of leukemia can vary depending on the type and stage of the disease but often include fatigue, weakness, frequent infections, enlarged lymph nodes, easy bleeding or bruising, weight loss, and bone or joint pain. However, these symptoms are not exclusive to leukemia and may also be associated with other conditions, so it's important to consult a healthcare professional for a proper diagnosis.

Diagnosis of leukemia typically involves a thorough medical history, physical examination, and blood tests to analyze the number and type of blood cells. Additional tests such as bone marrow biopsy, cytogenetic analysis, and molecular testing may also be performed to determine the specific type of leukemia and guide treatment decisions.

Treatment for leukemia depends on factors such as the type and stage of the disease, age, overall health, and individual preferences. Common treatment options include chemotherapy, targeted therapy, radiation therapy, immunotherapy, and stem cell transplantation. The goal of treatment is to destroy cancer cells, prevent the spread of the disease, and allow healthy blood cells to regenerate.

While leukemia can be a challenging and life-altering diagnosis, advancements in medical technology and treatment options have significantly improved the prognosis for many patients. Early detection, proper treatment, and ongoing care can help manage the disease and improve the quality of life for individuals with leukemia. It's important for patients to work closely with their healthcare team, seek support from loved ones and support groups, and follow recommended medical guidelines to optimize their well-being.

Leukemia is a type of cancer that starts in the bone marrow and affects the production of healthy blood cells. The exact causes of leukemia are still unknown, but there are several factors that have been associated with an increased risk of developing the disease. Here are some known factors:

CAUSES OF LEUKEMIA

1. Genetic Factors: Certain genetic mutations and chromosomal abnormalities have been linked to an increased risk of developing leukemia. These genetic changes can be inherited from parents or acquired over a person's lifetime.

2. Environmental Factors: Exposure to certain environmental factors has been associated with an increased risk of leukemia. These include exposure to high levels of ionizing radiation, such as medical radiation or atomic bomb radiation, exposure to certain chemicals like benzene, certain pesticides, and some

chemotherapy drugs used to treat other cancers.

3. Family History: People with a family history of leukemia have a slightly higher risk of developing the disease. However, most cases of leukemia occur in people without any family history of the disease.

4. Certain Medical Conditions: Some medical conditions are known to increase the risk of developing certain types of leukemia. For example, individuals with certain genetic disorders, such as Down syndrome, Fanconi anemia, or Li-Fraumeni syndrome, have a higher risk of developing leukemia.

5. Previous Cancer Treatment: Previous exposure to radiation or certain

chemotherapy drugs used to treat other types of cancer can increase the risk of developing leukemia later in life. This is known as secondary or treatment-related leukemia.

It's important to note that having one or more of these risk factors doesn't necessarily mean that a person will develop leukemia. In fact, most people with these risk factors never develop the disease. Additionally, many cases of leukemia occur in people without any known risk factors. The specific cause of leukemia can vary from person to person, and more research is needed to fully understand its origins.

PREVENTION OF LEUKEMIA

Leukemia is a type of cancer that affects the blood and bone marrow. While there is no surefire way to prevent leukemia, there are some strategies that may reduce the risk or help in early detection. Here are some prevention measures and lifestyle choices that can be considered:

1. Avoid exposure to certain chemicals and toxins: Limit exposure to chemicals like benzene, formaldehyde, and certain pesticides, as they have been linked to an increased risk of leukemia. Follow safety protocols if you work with potentially harmful substances and ensure your living environment is free from such toxins.

CANCER | Julius Iseman

2. Quit smoking: Smoking has been associated with various types of cancer, including leukemia. Quitting smoking and avoiding secondhand smoke can reduce your risk.

3. Protect yourself from radiation exposure: Minimize your exposure to ionizing radiation, such as excessive medical imaging tests or occupational exposure. Follow safety guidelines when undergoing X-rays, radiation therapy, or other radiation-based medical procedures.

4. Maintain a healthy lifestyle: Focus on adopting healthy habits, including a balanced diet rich in fruits, vegetables, and whole grains, regular exercise, and maintaining a healthy weight. These lifestyle choices can

help support general well-being and potentially reduce the risk of cancer, including leukemia.

5. Practice safe handling of chemotherapy drugs: If you work in a healthcare setting or are involved in handling chemotherapy drugs, take appropriate safety precautions to avoid exposure to these toxic substances.

6. Be aware of genetic predisposition: If you have a family history of leukemia or other types of cancer, it is important to discuss this with your healthcare provider. They may recommend genetic testing or specific screenings to monitor any potential risks.

7. Regular medical check-ups: Regular health check-ups can help in early detection and diagnosis. Discuss with your doctor about any concerns or symptoms you may have, ensuring that any underlying conditions are managed promptly.

It's important to note that leukemia can occur in individuals without any identifiable risk factors. While these preventive measures can help reduce certain risks, they are not foolproof. It is always advisable to consult with healthcare professionals for personalized guidance and to stay up-to-date with the latest medical research and recommendations regarding leukemia prevention.

CHAPTER 10

LYMPHOMA

Lymphoma is a type of cancer that originates in the lymphatic system, which is a part of the body's immune system. The lymphatic system consists of lymph nodes, lymphatic vessels, and lymphocytes (a type of white blood cell).

Lymphoma occurs when abnormal lymphocytes grow out of control and form tumors in the lymph nodes or other parts of the lymphatic system. There are two main types of lymphoma: Hodgkin lymphoma (HL) and non-Hodgkin lymphoma (NHL). These types differ in terms of the specific lymphocytes involved, the pattern of spread, and the overall prognosis.

Hodgkin lymphoma is characterized by the presence of Reed-Sternberg cells, large abnormal cells found in the lymph nodes. It typically starts in a single lymph node and may then spread to nearby nodes or other organs. Hodgkin lymphoma often has a predictable pattern of spread, with involvement of lymph node regions in a specific order. It is usually diagnosed at a younger age and has a good prognosis, with high cure rates, especially in earlier stages.

Non-Hodgkin lymphoma, on the other hand, comprises a large group of lymphomas that do not involve Reed-Sternberg cells. It is further categorized into various subtypes, each with its own unique characteristics. Non-Hodgkin lymphoma can develop in any lymphatic tissue and has a wider range of presentations and prognoses than Hodgkin lymphoma.

The exact causes of lymphoma are not fully understood, but certain factors may increase the likelihood of developing the disease. These include a weakened immune system, exposure to certain viruses (such as Epstein-Barr virus or human immunodeficiency virus), exposure to chemicals (such as herbicides or insecticides), and a family history of lymphoma.

Common symptoms of lymphoma may include swollen lymph nodes, weight loss, fever, night sweats, fatigue, and itching. However, symptoms can vary depending on the type and stage of lymphoma, and some people may not have any noticeable symptoms until the disease is more advanced.

Diagnosis of lymphoma involves a combination of medical history evaluation, physical examination, imaging tests (such as computed tomography or positron emission tomography scans), and biopsy of affected lymph nodes or other tissues. Additional laboratory tests may be performed to determine the specific type and extent of the lymphoma.

Treatment options for lymphoma depend on the type, stage, and characteristics of the disease. They can include chemotherapy, radiation therapy, immunotherapy, targeted therapy, or stem cell transplantation. The choice of treatment aims to eliminate or control the cancer cells while minimizing side effects.

Regular follow-ups and monitoring are often necessary after completing treatment for lymphoma to ensure any recurrence or late effects are detected early. Supportive care, including managing side effects and addressing emotional well-being, is also an important aspect of the overall management of lymphoma.

It's important to consult with a healthcare professional for an accurate diagnosis and personalized treatment plan if you suspect you may have lymphoma or are concerned about any symptoms you are experiencing. They can provide specific guidance tailored to your situation and help you navigate through the treatment process.

CAUSES OF LYMPHOMA

Lymphoma is a type of cancer that develops in the cells of the lymphatic system, which is a part of the body's immune system. The exact causes of lymphoma are not fully understood, but there are several factors that may contribute to its development. Here are some potential causes and risk factors associated with lymphoma:

1. Genetic predisposition: Certain genetic mutations or inherited conditions can increase the risk of developing lymphoma. For example, people with a family history of lymphoma are more likely to develop the disease.

2. Weakened immune system: Individuals with weak or compromised immune systems have a higher risk of developing lymphoma. This can be due to conditions such as HIV/AIDS,

certain autoimmune diseases, organ transplantation, or the use of immunosuppressive medications.

3. Infections: Some infections have been associated with an increased risk of lymphoma. The Epstein-Barr virus (EBV), which causes mononucleosis, is linked to certain types of lymphoma, such as Burkitt lymphoma and Hodgkin lymphoma. Other infections, such as hepatitis C virus (HCV) and human T-cell leukemia virus (HTLV-1), have also been implicated in the development of specific types of lymphoma.

4. Exposure to certain chemicals or substances: Prolonged exposure to certain chemicals and substances may increase the risk of lymphoma.

These include pesticides, herbicides (such as glyphosate), benzene (found in gasoline and chemical industries), and certain solvents.

5. Age and gender: Lymphoma can occur at any age, but the risk increases with age. Certain types of lymphoma, such as Hodgkin lymphoma, tend to affect young adults and children more often. Additionally, some types of lymphoma have a higher incidence in males, while others have a slightly higher incidence in females.

It is important to note that while these factors may increase the likelihood of developing lymphoma, not everyone exposed to them will develop the disease. Lymphoma is a complex condition, and additional research is needed to further understand its causes and risk factors. If you have concerns about lymphoma or any health-related issue, it is always recommended to consult with a medical professional for a thorough evaluation.

PREVENTION OF LYMPHOMA

The prevention of lymphoma generally focuses on reducing the risk factors associated with the development of the disease. It's important to note that, while some risk factors can be modified, others are beyond our control. Here are some strategies that may help lower the risk of developing lymphoma:

1. Stay physically active: Engage in regular exercise or physical activity

to maintain a healthy weight and overall well-being. Physical activity has been associated with a reduced risk of certain types of lymphoma.

2. Healthy diet: Follow a balanced diet that includes a variety of fruits, vegetables, whole grains, lean proteins, and healthy fats. Limit the consumption of processed foods, sugary drinks, and unhealthy fats. A nutritious diet supports a strong immune system.

3. Avoid tobacco and limit alcohol consumption: Smoking is strongly linked to an increased risk of various cancers, including some types of lymphoma. Likewise, excessive alcohol consumption has been associated with an increased risk of

CANCER | Julius Iseman

lymphoma. Avoiding tobacco and limiting alcohol intake is crucial for reducing the risk.

4. Protect against infections: Certain infections, such as the Epstein-Barr virus (EBV) and human T-cell lymphotropic virus (HTLV), have been linked to an increased risk of lymphoma. To prevent these infections, practice good hygiene, avoid sharing personal items with infected individuals, and practice safe sex.

5. Occupational and environmental exposure: Minimize exposure to known carcinogens and toxins in the workplace and the environment. If you work with chemicals or other potentially harmful substances,

ensure proper safety measures are in place and follow recommended protocols.

6. Prioritize immune system health: Maintain a healthy immune system by getting adequate sleep, managing stress, and practicing good hygiene. A strong immune system can help prevent infections and reduce the risk of lymphoma.

7. Regular medical check-ups: Attend routine medical check-ups to detect any potential health issues early. Follow recommended cancer screening guidelines, as some types of lymphoma can be detected in their early stages.

It's important to remember that while these strategies can help reduce the risk of

CANCER | Julius Iseman

lymphoma, they do not guarantee prevention. Additionally, some subtypes of lymphoma may have genetic or unknown causes, making prevention more challenging. If you have concerns about lymphoma risk factors, it's advisable to consult with a healthcare professional for personalized advice and guidance.

CHAPTER 11

BRAIN CANCER

Brain cancer, also known as brain tumors, refers to the abnormal and uncontrolled growth of cells in the brain. These cells form a mass or tumor, which can interfere with the normal functioning of the brain. Brain tumors can be classified as either benign (non-cancerous) or malignant (cancerous).

Malignant brain tumors are further categorized based on the type of cell they originated from within the brain. The most common type is a glioma, which develops from the glial cells that support and nourish the neurons. Other types include meningiomas (originating from the meninges), metastatic tumors (cancers that have spread to the brain from other parts of the body), and others.

Brain cancer can cause a wide range of symptoms depending on its size and location. Some common symptoms include headaches, seizures, changes in vision or hearing, difficulties with speech or movement, memory problems, personality changes, and unexplained nausea or vomiting. However, these symptoms are not specific to brain cancer and can also be caused by other conditions.

The exact cause of brain cancer is often unknown, although certain risk factors can increase the likelihood of developing it. These include exposure to ionizing radiation, certain inherited gene mutations, a history of certain hereditary conditions, and a family history of brain tumors. However, most individuals with these risk factors do not develop brain cancer, and many cases occur in individuals without any known risk factors.

The diagnosis of brain cancer typically involves imaging tests such as MRI or CT scans, which provide detailed pictures of the brain. A biopsy, where a small sample of the tumor is removed for analysis, is often needed to determine the type and grade of the tumor. Treatment options vary depending on factors such as the type, size, location, and grade of the tumor, as well as the overall health of the patient. Treatment may involve surgery, radiation therapy, chemotherapy, targeted therapy, or a combination of these approaches.

The prognosis for brain cancer depends on various factors, including the type and stage of the tumor, its location, the age and overall health of the individual, and the treatment received. Some brain tumors can be successfully treated, especially if they are low-grade and located in accessible areas. However, others can be more aggressive and difficult to treat, leading to poorer outcomes. It is important to consult with a medical professional for accurate diagnosis, individualized treatment plans, and ongoing support.

CAUSES OF BRAIN CANCER

Brain cancer, also known as brain tumors, can originate from different types of cells within the brain, including glial cells, neurons, and others. While the exact causes of brain cancer are not always clear, several factors are known to be potential contributors to its development. Here are some recognized causes and risk factors associated with brain cancer:

1. Genetic factors: Certain inherited gene mutations can increase the risk of developing brain tumors. These genetic abnormalities are relatively rare, but individuals with certain genetic conditions such as neurofibromatosis, Li-Fraumeni syndrome, tuberous sclerosis, von Hippel-Lindau disease, and others have a higher chance of developing brain cancer.

2. Exposure to radiation: Exposure to ionizing radiation, either from medical procedures like radiation

therapy to treat previous cancers or from environmental factors such as nuclear accidents or radiation-emitting devices, may increase the risk of brain cancer in some individuals.

3. Age: Brain cancer can affect people of all ages, but certain types, such as glioblastoma multiforme, tend to occur more frequently in older adults.

4. Family history: While most brain tumors are not hereditary, having a family history of brain cancer can slightly increase the risk.

5. Exposure to certain chemicals: Occupational exposure to certain chemicals, such as vinyl chloride and formaldehyde, has been associated with an increased risk of brain cancer.

 CANCER | Julius Iseman

However, the majority of brain tumors do not have a clear link to specific chemical exposures.

6. Immune system disorders: Some studies suggest that individuals with weakened immune systems due to conditions like HIV/AIDS or those who have received organ transplants may have an elevated risk of developing brain cancer.

It is important to note that in the majority of cases, the exact cause of brain cancer remains unknown, and many people diagnosed with brain tumors do not have any identifiable risk factors. If you have concerns about brain cancer, it is advisable to consult with a healthcare professional who can provide personalized information and guidance based on your specific situation.

PREVENTION OF BRAIN CANCER

The prevention of brain cancer involves a combination of lifestyle choices, environmental factors, and early detection. While there is no guaranteed way to prevent brain cancer, the following steps can help reduce the risk:

1. Maintain a Healthy Lifestyle: Adopting a healthy lifestyle can contribute to overall well-being, including reducing the risk of cancer. This includes regularly engaging in physical activity, eating a balanced diet rich in fruits, vegetables, and whole grains, limiting processed

foods and red meat consumption, and avoiding excessive alcohol consumption or tobacco use.

2. Protect Against Radiation: Exposure to ionizing radiation is a known risk factor for brain cancer. Minimize unnecessary exposure to radiation by following safety guidelines and minimizing exposure to sources like X-rays, CT scans, and radiation therapy unless medically necessary.

3. Protect Against Carcinogens: Some environmental factors and occupational exposures can increase the risk of brain cancer. Limit exposure to potential carcinogens, such as hazardous chemicals, pesticides, and other industrial toxins. Follow safety guidelines at work and

use appropriate protective equipment if necessary.

4. Protect Against Viral Infections: Certain viral infections, such as human immunodeficiency virus (HIV) and certain types of herpes virus, have been associated with an increased risk of developing brain cancer. Taking preventive measures against these viruses, such as practicing safe sex, getting vaccinated for relevant diseases, and maintaining a healthy immune system, may help reduce the risk.

5. Wear Protective Headgear: Taking precautions to protect your head can lower the risk of traumatic brain injuries, which have been linked to the development of brain cancer. For

example, while participating in high-risk activities or certain sports, wear appropriate helmets or headgear to minimize the risk of head injuries.

6. Regular Medical Check-ups: Regular check-ups with your healthcare provider can help identify any early symptoms or warning signs related to brain cancer. Prompt medical attention can lead to early detection, potentially improving treatment outcomes.

Remember that these measures can reduce the risk of developing brain cancer, but they do not guarantee complete prevention. If you have concerns about brain cancer or any other health issues, it's important to consult with a healthcare professional for personalized advice and guidance.

CONCLUSION

In conclusion, cancer is a complex and multifaceted disease with significant impact on individuals, families, and societies worldwide. It is characterized by the uncontrolled growth and spread of abnormal cells, which can occur in various parts of the body. Cancer manifests in numerous types, each presenting distinct characteristics and treatment approaches.

Over the years, significant progress has been made in understanding cancer's causes, risk factors, and mechanisms. Genetic mutations, environmental factors, lifestyle choices, and viral infections can contribute to the development of cancer. Early detection, screening, and improved diagnostic techniques have allowed for better prognosis and treatment outcomes.

The treatment of cancer often involves a multidisciplinary approach, combining surgery, chemotherapy, radiation therapy, targeted therapy, and immunotherapy. Personalized medicine is also gaining prominence, tailoring treatments based on a patient's specific genetic profile and tumor characteristics.

Despite advancements, cancer remains a significant global health issue, causing immense suffering and mortality. It is essential to continually invest in research, prevention strategies, and access to quality healthcare to reduce cancer incidence and improve survival rates. Public awareness campaigns, education, and lifestyle modifications play a crucial role in reducing cancer risks, promoting early detection, and improving overall well-being.

CANCER | Julius Iseman

Efforts to alleviate the burden of cancer include global initiatives, collaborations between researchers, and the development of innovative therapies. These endeavors aim to improve patient outcomes, enhance quality of life during treatment, and ultimately find a cure for cancer.

Although there is still much work to be done, the collective efforts of healthcare professionals, researchers, policy-makers, and society as a whole provide hope for a future free from the devastation caused by cancer. With continued progress, cancer prevention, early detection, and effective treatment will contribute to improving the lives of those affected by this disease and ultimately contribute to a healthier world.

Cancer, one of the most formidable diseases known to humanity, has captivated the attention of scientists, medical professionals, and individuals worldwide. It is a complex and multifaceted condition characterized by the uncontrolled growth and spread of abnormal cells in the body. This ailment has a profound impact on individuals, families, and societies, making it an ongoing challenge in the field of healthcare.

Cancer can manifest in various forms, affecting different organs and systems within the body. It arises from genetic mutations that alter the normal behavior of cells, leading to their unrestrained division and proliferation. These mutations can be caused by a variety of factors, including environmental influences such as exposure to harmful substances, lifestyle choices like smoking or excessive sun exposure, or even inherent genetic predispositions.

The repercussions of cancer extend beyond the mere presence of abnormal cells. As the disease progresses, it can infiltrate nearby tissues, impair vital organ function, and ultimately spread to distant sites in a process known as metastasis. This invasive nature of cancer poses significant challenges for treatment and management, as it requires comprehensive and personalized approaches to combat the disease effectively.

The impact of cancer reaches far beyond the physical toll it takes on the body. It affects individuals emotionally, mentally, and socially, often causing distress, fear, and uncertainty. Moreover, cancer can strain relationships, disrupt daily routines, and impose financial burdens on those affected. The profound psychological and emotional implications highlight the need for comprehensive support systems and holistic care for cancer patients, as their journey involves not only medical interventions but also psychological and emotional well-being.

Fortunately, immense strides have been made in cancer research over the years. Advances in technology, diagnostics, and treatments have significantly improved outcomes for many patients. New therapies such as targeted therapies, immunotherapies, and precision medicine have revolutionized the field, offering hope for those affected by the disease. Moreover, preventive measures such as early detection screenings and lifestyle modifications have proven effective in reducing the risk of developing certain types of cancer.

The understanding and management of cancer continue to evolve, with ongoing research striving to unlock its mysteries.

Collaboration between scientists, clinicians, and advocacy groups has played a pivotal role in raising awareness, funding research, and improving outcomes. Efforts to enhance public knowledge about prevention, screening, and early detection are essential in reducing the impact of cancer.

Finally, cancer remains a significant global health concern, posing complex challenges for medical professionals, researchers, and society as a whole. It demands continuous progress in diagnosis, treatment, and support systems to alleviate its burden. Although the battle against cancer is far from over, the collective efforts of healthcare professionals, researchers, and individuals affected by this disease provide hope for a future where cancer is better understood, controlled, and ultimately cured.